ANCIENT MEDICINE

by Dr. Desmond Corrigan

B.Sc (Pharmacy), M.A., Ph.D., F.L.S., F.P.S.I.

Published by
Amberwood Publishing Ltd
Park Corner, Park Horsley, East Horsley, Surrey KT24 5RZ
Tel: 01483 285919

ISBN 0-9517723-4-1

Typeset and designed by
Word Perfect, Christchurch, Dorset.

Cover design by Design Hive

Printed in Great Britain

CONTENTS

About the Author

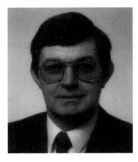

Senior Lecturer and Head
of the Department of
Pharmacognosy,
School of Pharmacy,
University of Dublin,
Trinity College, Ireland.

Dr. Corrigan was born and educated in Dublin. After obtaining his degree in Pharmacy he spent some time in the pharmaceutical industry before joining the staff of the School of Pharmacy. Dr. Corrigan is a former analyst with the Drug Squad of the Irish Police and since 1980 he has been deeply involved in community drug education and other drug prevention activities. He is author of "Facts about Drug Abuse in Ireland", now in its Third Edition. Dr. Corrigan's research is concentrated in the area of phytotherapy, in particular, aspects of the quality control of phytomedicines and the testing of herbal medicines used by a traditional Irish herbalist. Dr. Corrigan has lectured at many national and international conferences on phyto-therapy. He is co-chairman of the Scientific Committee of ESCOP - the European Scientific Cooperative on Phyto-therapy - and a member of the Editorial Advisory Boards of the International Journal of Pharmacognosy, of the British Journal of Phytotherapy and of the European Journal of Herbal Medicine.

Listed among his hobbies are good wines, travel, political thrillers, history and light classical music.

Introduction

The Planet Earth along with its human, its animal and its plant life has seen many significant, often cataclysmic events, during the millions of years it has existed. One such earth shattering event took place on August 6th 1945 at 8.15am local time above the Japanese city of Hiroshima when the first atomic bomb exploded. An incredible flash of light followed by a sudden wave of intense heat led to the now familiar mushroom cloud extending to 40,000 feet. In its wake nearly 4 square miles of the city were completely devastated with over 66,000 of its inhabitants killed, another 69,000 injured and over two-thirds of the city's structures destroyed or severely damaged.

Out of all of that death and destruction, one tree survived to push up new green shoots, so that today a Ginkgo tree flourishes in what was virtually the centre of that nuclear explosion. It is not surprising that the Ginkgo tree should have survived one of mankind's most destructive acts because Ginkgo could be labelled the Great Survivor since this "living fossil" first appeared on the earth some 190 million years ago and it has survived all the changes which have taken place since then. What is surprising is that this oldest of living plants should be still yielding up its secrets to medical science – secrets which are already bringing relief to large numbers-of patients and which could, in the future, bring relief to sufferers of conditions as diverse as asthma, transplant rejection, cerebral insufficiency, shock and stroke.

This book is a voyage of discovery of Ginkgo from its origins in a world inhabited by dinosaurs to the unique properties of the medicines which are made from its leaves. It looks at the tree, its unique ability to act as a chemical factory, at the medicinal properties of the chemicals it produces and at the efforts to bring those properties to the frail, the elderly and the ill, who will benefit most from the partnership of modern science and ancient medicinal plant.

Note to Reader

Whilst the author has made every effort to ensure that the contents of this book are accurate in every particular, it is not intended to be regarded as a substitute for professional medical advice under treatment. The reader is urged to give careful consideration to any difficulties which he or she is experiencing with their own health and to consult their General Practitioner if uncertain as to its cause or nature. Neither the author nor the publisher can accept any legal responsibility for any health problem which results from use of the self-help methods described.

Publisher's Note

In the light of some new and remarkable research concerning the benefits of 'Ginkgo', the publishers and author have produced this updated edition. For those of you who are familiar with the original text, or those who have a particular interest, please note that the changes and additions are as follows:

Original text, addition: "Other effects' – Re Multiple Sclerosis, page 31.

Original text, addition: 'Ginkgo and Intermittent Claudication' – Re Meta-analysis as to the effect of Ginkgo in clinical trials, page 35.

Original text, additional evidence on safety, page 41.

New section, page 36: Vertigo and Sudden Deafness.

New section, page 36: Pre-menstrual Syndrome

New section, page 37: Ginkgo and Subarachnoid Haemorrhage.

1 | The Ginkgo Story – of Dinosaurs and Men

When Ginkgo and its ancestors first appeared on the Earth, the planet was a very different place to the Earth we know today. Plant life was dominated by giant horsetails and ferns but there were no grasses or trees. There were no mammals, only dinosaurs, and their precursors, the thecodants, as well as mammal-like reptiles, the therapsids. The first real trees appeared about 250-700 million years ago and included relatives of what we now call *Ginkgo biloba*. The cold weather and physical action of the glaciers during the Ice Age 2 million years ago led to the extinction of many plant species including all of the Ginkgo species except *G. biloba*, which apparently escaped when the ice stopped its relentless progression in Eastern Asia. The Ginkgo trees of today appear to be essentially unchanged from their ancestors which have been discovered as fossils in Asia, Europe, America, Argentina and Australia. Because of the similarity between the fossil Ginkgos and the living plant, Ginkgo is usually referred to as a "living fossil" which has probably existed on Earth longer than any other tree. We are fortunate that it continued to exist in the warm-temperate forests of China where it was eventually discovered by humans. The wild populations are believed to have become extinct thousands of years ago and the tree is believed to have survived only because of human intervention because of its valuable fruit, its wood and its medicinal value and possibly because of an appreciation of its intrinsic beauty by Buddhist monks who planted it around their temples.

The Ginkgo Tree

It is undoubtedly a beautiful tree, with its fan-shaped leaves (hence the name "maidenhair tree") and its fruits, referred to by the Chinese as Silver Apricots. Throughout Asia there are many large and ancient specimens of Ginkgo that are over 1000 years old. The tree can grow to a height of over 30 metres and has reached a breadth of 7 metres. The tree has a grey coloured bark. The plant produces two types of branches resulting in long and short shoots. Leaves grow along the whole of the long shoot and as clusters at the ends of both the long and short shoots each spring. The leaves are a light green colour when young turning to a deep green colour when mature and a golden yellow colour in Autumn. The leaves are leathery, fan shaped and frequently deeply bilobed hence the botanical name given to the plant by the Swedish botanist, Linnaeus in 1771 when he called the tree *Ginkgo biloba*. The wood of the tree is soft, straight-grained with a light brown colour and a silky sheen and it has the ability to repel insects. This wood has been used commercially to manufacture small cabinets, abacus beads, chessmen, seals and fine oriental lacquer wares [Staba 1992].

Under conditions of moderate soil fertility, Ginkgo grows quickly, averaging between 30-50cms per year. Sexual maturity is reached when the tree is 20-30 years old and height growth slows at this stage as the tree broadens and begins to produce sexual organs. Ginkgo is described as a dioecious plant species, that is, the male and female flowers are produced on separate trees. Hermaphrodite Ginkgo trees have been rarely observed. The reproductive organs appear on trees that are at least 20 years old, producing seeds with a fleshy outer layer which emits a foul odour making the female plant which bears the seeds less desirable as an ornamental plant.

Ginkgo in Cultivation

There is considerable doubt as to whether any wild Ginkgo trees still exist. Some Chinese botanists believe that wild trees existed in China as late as 1933, but it is widely believed that human intervention has saved ginkgo from extinction because of a recognition of its value as a food, an ornamental and as a medicine. Indeed it was as valued as Ginseng during the Sung dynasty [late 10th Century] in China, the seeds being sent as a yearly tribute to the Emperor. Records show that it was planted in the capital city, Kaifeng, at that time. It is not known when exactly it was introduced into Japan but trees were observed in 1690 in Japan by Kaempfer, a Dutch surgeon. The species was subsequently brought to Europe in 1730 and into England in 1754. The first recorded ginkgo trees in America were those planted in Philadelphia in 1784. Ginkgo is now cultivated extensively in Asia, Europe, North America and the temperate regions of New Zealand and Argentina.

Ginkgo grows well in most parts of the world where there are distinct seasons and moderate rainfall. This includes areas with the typical Mediterranean climate, i.e. wet, mild winters and hot dry summers as well as those with a cold climate where the temperature can drop as low as −20°. While it grows best in full sunlight it can also flourish in conditions of low light such as the downtown streets of many skyscraper-dominated American cities. The reason for its popularity for urban planting in the U.S. stems from its great power of survival as well as its higher degree of resistance to insects and to fungal, viral and bacterial disease compared to other cultivated trees. In the earlier part of this century horticulturists believed that it was highly tolerant of air pollution from burning coal but it does not seem to be any more immune to ozone and sulphur dioxide that any other tree. When the unpleasant smell of the fruits and their skin irritant effects were noted in the 1920's and 30's there was less enthusiasm for the tree as an ornamental but it has always been widely cultivated in China both as an ornamental around imperial palaces and in Japan around Buddhist temples. Many of the magnificent specimens which can be seen in Japan, China and Korea are believed to be over 1000 years old.

The reason for its longevity is a mystery, but it possesses an extraordinary ability to adapt to a huge variety of environments. At one time it was believed to be immune to the chromosome damaging effects of radiation and this was believed to explain why the famous tree in Hiroshima survived. However the truth is that it is as susceptible to radiation as any other tree but because Ginkgo takes so long [20years] to start reproducing, genetic damage may be reduced.

Whatever about its resistance, or lack of it, to radiation, Ginkgo is remarkably resistant to pest and diseases, due to the chemicals that it produces in various parts of the tree as a means of defence. For example, extracts of the leaves and roots prevent the growth of the Cabbage Butterfly caterpillar and other insects. Leaf extracts also prevent the growth of many bacteria, while root compounds prevent certain virus diseases of plants. The importance of these chemical constituents cannot be over-stressed since they have in all probability been responsible for the survival of this unique living fossil for over 200 million years. This ability to survive the ravages of time, pollution and pests may have a message for us humans in that it might, à la Doctrine of Signatures, be telling us that Ginkgo while in no way being the Elixir of Youth, could help us withstand some of the difficulties caused by the ravages of time.

Ginkgo as a Traditional Medicine

The use of Ginkgo as a human medicine dates back almost 5000 years. It is mentioned in the oldest of the Chinese herbals, the Shen Nuong Ben Cao Jing, written about 2800BC. Subsequently it featured in many of the major Chinese herbals, for example, in the Dian Nan Ben Cao by Lan Mao during the Ming dynasty and dated around 1436AD. This "Pharmaceutical Natural History of Southern Yunnan" recommended the external use of the leaves to treat skin and head sores as well as freckles. The first mention of the internal use of the plant came in the Ben Cao Pin Hue Jing Yao [Essentials of the Pharmacopoeia ranked according to

Nature and Efficacy], a work commissioned by the imperial court recorded in 1505. The author Liu Wen-tai noted the use of the leaves in the treatment of diarrhoea.

The great Chinese herbal, the Pen Ts'ao Kan Mu, by Li Shih-Chen which first saw the light of day in 1595 discussed the origin and names of Ginkgo and included an illustration of the foliage and fruit. The plant also appears in the Herbal for Food by Li Tung Wan and the Herbal for Daily Usage by Wu Jui both of which appeared in the 14th Century. The leaves known in Traditional Chinese Medicine as "Bai-gui-ye" have been used to treat asthma and coughs. They are also reported to "benefit the brain" and have been used in the treatment of the parasitic disease filariasis. Modern Chinese Medicine uses tablets and injections of Ginkgo in the treatment of angina, chronic bronchitis and to lower serum cholesterol levels. A tea made from the leaves is used in the treatment of frost bite. As we will see in the following chapters, modern scientific research has shown that many of these traditional indications for using the plant are based on a fairly solid basis. In traditional Hindu medicine, Ginkgo is reported as a constituent of the Soma elixir.

Nowadays Ginkgo is extensively cultivated on a commercial basis in China for its seeds or nuts which are a prized delicacy and in Europe and the U.S.A. for its formidable medicinal properties.

Ginkgo Seeds

Traditionally Ginkgo seeds were used as a food in Asia and to aid digestion and to reduce the intoxicating effects of wine, which is perhaps why Japanese bars serve the pale green nuts as a tasty accompaniment to cold beer. Cosmetics and soaps have been prepared from the seed and the outer fleshy layer of the seed. These seeds usually fall from the tree two-three weeks after the leaves. At first they have only a faint odour but after a few days the outer layer starts to decompose giving rise to an unpleasant rancid odour described in the horticultural literature as "disagreeable", "offensive" and "repulsive". The reason for the disgusting smell is a mixture of fatty acids such as formic, butyric and caproic acids among others. The fleshy part of the seed has also been reported to raise welts on the skin of both humans and rabbits in patch tests. Extracts have been found to contain a phenolic compound, ginkgolic acid, which is the compound responsible for this allergic reaction. It is chemically similar to anacardic acid, the toxic compound found in the Cashew Nut tree.

Inside the ginkgo seed is the hard shelled, edible nut which is highly nutritious containing 37% carbohydrate, 4% protein, 1.7% fat and yields 1.8 calories per gram. Most of the carbohydrate is starch, but small amounts of sucrose, glucose and fructose give the nut a sweet taste.

Asian horticulturists have focused their attention on the cultivation of the tree for those edible nuts. The Chinese have developed at least 28 varieties based on the size and shape of the nut. The seeds are processed to allow the smelly part to be washed away, after which they are dried in the air and stored in a cool place.

The seed must be cooked for human consumption. The kernels can be removed to make a sweet soup or they can be pan fried and then eaten. They have a flavour like those of the sweet chestnut but excessive consumption of more than seven nuts at one time is considered inadvisable due to toxic side-effects. Ginkgo nuts are considered an Asian delicacy and can fetch up to $1.50 per kilo. Supplies from the estimated five million kilograms of seed produced each year in China are sent to Chinese people living in other parts of Asia, in Europe and in North America.

Cultivation as a Medicinal Plant

More recent interest in growing ginkgo has stemmed from the enormous interest in it as a medicine in Europe where sales of Ginkgo products amount to at least $500 million a year. Large scale plantations specifically for the purpose of medicine extraction were established near Bordeaux in France and in Sumter, South Carolina, in 1982. In Sumter there are some 10 million specially pruned trees planted on 400 hectares [1,000 acres]. Harvesting of the leaves is performed mechanically from mid-August to mid-September yielding about 4,000 kilograms of dried leaves per hectare. After drying to reduce moisture content to 12 percent, the leaves are packed in 180 kilogram bales, taken to Charleston, South Carolina, and then shipped to the extraction plants in Europe where the chemicals developed over millions of years are removed for use in human medicines.

2 | The Chemistry of Ginkgo – of Sun, C and Sex

During the oil shortages and crises of the 1970's and 80's we heard much about the need to use solar energy as an alternative source of power. We tend to ignore the fact that as humans we are uniquely dependent on solar energy for our continued existence on this planet. The food we eat and the oxygen we breathe are produced for us as a result of the hyper-efficient use of solar energy by the Plant Kingdom.

Plants use solar energy or sunlight to power the astonishing chemical factories found in each and every one of their cells. This chemical synthesis has its origins in the green chlorophyll-containing parts of the plant. Chlorophyll is the means by which plants can chemically combine solar energy, the small amounts of carbon dioxide in air and water from the soil, to produce usable food in the form of sugars. These represent, in essence, energy trapped from sunlight in the process of photosynthesis. A large number of the chemicals produced as a result of this most fundamental of life-giving chemical processes are essential to the existence of the plant and are common to most plants whatever their shape or size. These chemicals are usually referred to as products of primary metabolism and include materials such as the carbohydrates (the 'C' of the chapter heading), the lipids or fats and the proteins. In addition, most plants produce other chemicals which may be unique to that one plant or they may be found in a group of plants. The function of these compounds, called **secondary metabolites**, is often not fully understood, but may, as in the case of the Ginkgo chemicals, be responsible for the ability of the plant to protect itself against predators and disease.

Secondary metabolism is not a distinct process but rather a continuation of primary metabolism using chemicals produced during, for example, photosynthesis as starting materials. One of the most remarkable features of this process is that plants use just three very simple materials to produce a vast range of complex chemicals, some of which cannot yet be synthesised in the laboratory. Many of these secondary metabolites are used as drugs in modern medicines, e.g. Digoxin for heart disease from the Foxglove, Morphine for pain from the Opium Poppy, Vincristine for leukaemia from the Madagascan Periwinkle. Others are responsible for the beneficial effects of the plants used in modern phytotherapy, e.g.

Ginseng, Feverfew, Agnus Castus, Valerian, Chamomile etc. The phenomenal capacity of even the simplest of plants to act as a sophisticated chemical laboratory is frequently underestimated and often ignored.

That criticism cannot be levelled at the many research groups who have investigated the phytochemistry [plant chemistry] of *Ginkgo biloba*. At the last count over 140 different chemical compounds have been isolated and identified in all parts of the plant. Some of these are responsible for the flavour of the seed, some are responsible for the plant's ability to defend itself against predators and disease, while others are bringing relief and comfort to thousands and thousands of human patients. The two key groups of secondary chemicals produced in the cells by the Ginkgo plant are the phenolics and the terpenoids.

Plant Phenolics

The phenols, so-called because of their chemical relationship to the disinfectant Phenol, constitute one of the largest groups of natural chemicals. Plants, bacteria and fungi have the ability to produce this type of six-carbon compounds, in contrast to animals who must consume pre-formed phenolics in the diet. Two types of Phenolics are important in Ginkgo, firstly the ginkgolic acids which are the irritant chemicals in the fleshy part of the fruit. More important are a group of phenolics called the **flavonoids**. Many people come in contact with flavonoids every day of their lives, because some flavonoid derivatives are responsible for the white, yellow, blue and red colours of flower petals. We consume large quantities of flavonoids in fruit and vegetables and in beverages such as tea and in particular red wine. There are about 2000 different flavonoids known to science and Ginkgo contains representatives of 5 separate groups including some biflavones [dimers containing two flavonoid molecules chemically joined together] and a group of flavonol glycosides where the phenolic structure is chemically linked to a sugar such as glucose. A 1993 report on the analysis of dried Ginkgo leaves from the commercial market shows that they contain between 0.5 to 1% by weight of flavonol glycosides. While the green leaves are considered to be of higher quality, research has shown that as far as the flavonoids are concerned it does not matter whether the leaves are harvested in June or November.

For many years all commercially available Ginkgo preparations were standardised on the "Ginkgo flavone glycoside content". Some enriched extracts contain 24% by weight, others between 1-6 and 25% . When these extracts are incorporated into tablets or liquid preparations, the content of flavonoids will be diluted so that they in fact are often comparable in content to products containing unprocessed plant material.

More recently Ginkgo products have been also standardised on their content of the second main group of chemicals, namely the terpene lactones.

Terpenes

Terpenes are another important group of plant chemicals. The story of their production starts with a biochemical form of acetic acid (which is more familiar to most of us as vinegar). Much of our knowledge of how plant and animal cells produce terpenes comes from studies of the production of cholesterol and rubber, both of which are natural terpenes. All terpenes are made from the same basic building block, a five carbon compound called isoprene. In the cell isoprene is found in a highly reactive form which undergoes a series of chemical reactions where several isoprene units are linked together as shown in the following scheme:

2 Biological Isoprene Units → Monoterpenes, e.g. menthol
[B.I.U.]   [10 carbons]   essential or
  ↓   volatile oils used
    in Gerard House
    Aromatherapy
    Range

  +1.[B.I.U.]
  ↓

Bilobalide   ← Sesquiterpenes
  [15 carbons]
[*active compound in Ginkgo*]   +1.[B.I.U.]
  ↓

Ginkgolides   ← Diterpenes
[*active compounds in Ginkgo*]   [20 carbons]
  ↓

  Triterpenes   →   Cholesterol
  Polyterpenes   →   Rubber

The ginkgolides are characteristic compounds of Ginkgo and indeed are specific to this plant. They are incredibly complex, incorporating six 5-membered rings in a chemically unique cage structure. [The prurient may like to be reminded that the latin for six is sex, hence the chapter subtitle!] As a recent review so neatly puts it "while *Ginkgo biloba* achieves total synthesis of ginkgolides with great ease, the synthesis of these compounds in the laboratory has provided one of the most formidable challenges to modern organic chemistry" [Braquet and Hosford, 1991].

In fact the total laboratory synthesis of one ginkgolide – ginkgolide B was only achieved in 1988 although the compounds themselves were first isolated as bitter compounds in 1932. The chemical structures were not established until the late 1960's. At the present time five distinct natural ginkgolides are known: Ginkgolides A, B, C, J and M (for minor) as well as some semisynthetic derivatives. The world-renowned Japanese chemist, Nakanishi, who elucidated the structures reports that the best source of ginkgolides is the root bark. Unfortunately this cannot be collected without destroying trees. [As a result of a typhoon, however, Nakanishi gained access to 100 kilos of root bark from 5 fallen trees in Sendai, Japan, from which he extracted 10 grams each of Ginkgolide A and B, 10 grams of Ginkgolide C and only 200 milligrammes of Ginkgolide M.]

Commercially the leaves are used as a source of the ginkgolides even though the concentration is fairly low – often below 0.1% by weight. Large differences in ginkgolide concentration have been reported in the scientific literature. There can be a 160 fold difference between the content at the end of October when it is highest and the content in young leaves. A 1993 study found that the ginkgolide and bilobalide content of Ginkgo leaves was highest in leaves from France [0.26%] and lowest in leaves from Holland [0.006%]. Bilobalide, a terpene containing 15 carbons, technically referred to as a sesquiterpene, could be detected during the whole growing season but its concentration was lowest in Spring, reached a maximum in mid-Summer and started to decline when the leaves turned yellow at the end of Autumn. Similar results are found with the Ginkgolides. However there can be significant differences between individual trees and it is apparent that this difference is far more important than the time of harvest. It is not known why these large differences exist. They could be due to the sex of the tree because there are reports that a male tree contained no detectable amounts of Ginkgolide B (the most active of the compounds). The differences could also be due to soil composition or the existence of what are called "chemical races" i.e. plants which are identical botanically but which differ significantly in their chemical composition. This is an area under active investigation at present.

As we will discover in the next chapter, the **flavonoids, the bilobalide** and the **ginkgolides**, all have starring roles in the story of how mankind is benefitting from this most unusual plant and how the marriage of modern science and ancient medicine is signposting new exciting medicines for many life-threatening diseases.

3 | Of Oxygen, Old Age and Arachidonic Acid

The story was told in the previous chapter of how plants trap energy from sunlight and convert it into food via carbon dioxide and water. Humans do the reverse. The food we eat is combined with oxygen and broken down to give back carbon dioxide, water and energy. This energy is used to run our bodies. The focus of a large part of our energy production is our brain. Even though it accounts for only about 2% of the total weight of the body, the human brain must receive about one-fifth of the body's total supply of blood and about one-fifth of our energy intake.

The human brain has to be that greedy because it cannot store either oxygen or energy and depends on an uninterrupted supply of a pint and a half of blood containing food and oxygen flowing through it every minute. Even a 10-second break in this supply can lead to unconsciousness. After about three minutes without blood supply, irreparable damage occurs. If the supply is cut for more than eight minutes then death is inevitable. Any insufficient blood supply to any part of the body is known medically as **ischaemia** and the resulting reduction of oxygen is referred to as **hypoxia**. Since nerve cells have a very high energy requirement to allow them function, they actually die if oxygen is not made available constantly to them.

Cerebral Ischaemia

The most important type of ischaemia is cerebral ischaemia, i.e. a loss or drastic reduction in blood flow to the cerebrum which is the main upper part of the brain consisting of two cerebral hemispheres, joined together. The cerebral cortex is the outer surface layer and contains the areas in which memory, intellect and emotion exist; movement and speech initiated; vision and sensation experienced, speech understood and creative activity undertaken.

Because of the importance of a continual blood supply to the brain the rest of the body could be considered as simply a way of supporting the brain and carrying out its decisions. The heart in particular must maintain the supply of blood to the brain through the arteries. The key arteries to the brain are the carotid and the vertebral arteries. Trouble arises if these arteries are diseased, particularly if they are affected by atherosclerosis. This is a combination of arteriosclerosis, i.e. hardening of what once was flexible elastic tubing taking the blood from the heart all through the body, added to a condition called atheroma.

As a result, fatty material is laid down on the inner lining of arteries so that they not only become narrowed but they are also liable to have the blood within them start to clot. If this clot blocks the artery where it is originally formed we have what is called a thrombosis, e.g. a coronary thrombosis where one of the arteries feeding the pumping muscles of the heart is blocked. Sometimes pieces of a clot break away and are carried in the blood stream. This material is called an embolus and may cause a blockage in an artery away from where it was originally formed. Emboli can be of different types of material. Some may be made up of fibrin and tiny blood cells called platelets, both of which are essential for blood clotting. Some may be formed from 'porridge'-like plaques of fat which constitute the artherosclerosis on the inside of arteries. The third type of embolism consists of pure crystals of cholesterol. Such embolisms are a common cause of stroke.

Stroke

The symptoms of stroke are very varied because any function of the brain can be affected if blood supply is impaired. The most obvious affects are weakness on one side of the body, numbness, disturbances of speech and understanding and visual problems. Less common are vertigo, nausea and vomiting, headache, loss of hearing and memory, gradual changes in personality and intellect, drowsiness, loss of consciousness and occasionally epileptic fits. A stroke is a dramatic and life-threatening event which obviously constitutes a full-scale medical emergency and involves hospitalisation and appropriate medical and surgical care.

Dementias

However, many people have a series of small indetectable strokes which occur over a period of time leaving clusters of dead nerve cells behind. Such small localised clusters of dead or damaged cells are known as infarcts and the resulting condition is known as Multiple Infarct Dementia or MID. MID reduces an individual's mental and social capabilities, affecting speech, judgement, emotions, coordination and common sense. There is a strong similarity between Multiple Infarct Dementia and another well-known type of dementia – Alzheimer's

Dementia (AD). MID can be distinguished from AD by the fact that MID generally affects people aged between 40-60 years, while AD doesn't usually show up until about age 65.

It has been estimated that about 7% of the 7 million people in Great Britain aged over 65 suffer from senile dementia. The symptoms include memory impairment, slowed movement and thought, confusion, amnesia, disorientation lethargy and paranoia

People with senile dementia lose brain cells at a much faster rate than normal and in some cases the ability of the nerve cells to work is damaged when they become entangled with strands of protein. Of those suffering from dementia, about half are believed to have Alzheimer's disease, another 20-30% may have a combination of Alzheimer's and MID, while the remainder suffer from MID alone.

Many other elderly people show evidence of intellectual impairment indicating that their brains may not be receiving an adequate supply of blood and hence oxygen and that they can no longer compensate for the normal loss of brain cells which takes place daily once we reach the age of about 20.

The formation of blood clots is a key event leading to the development of what is often called cerebral insufficiency The formation of a clot is the result of a complex series of events. A significant participant in these events is a tiny microscopic blood cell called a **platelet** (because it is normally plate-shaped). They can also be called **thrombocytes** because of their role in thrombosis or clotting. Normally, of course, your blood doesn't clot except when you cut yourself. With a cut you bleed for a few minutes then a clot is formed which plugs the wound and stops any further flow of blood. This clot is produced because your platelets have stuck together (aggregated) at the site of the injury. Additional platelets then stick to those already present and a complicated series of chemical reactions are activated within each platelet.

An enzyme (a protein which speeds up chemical reactions) causes part of the outer layer of the platelet to break off in the form of a fatty acid called Arachidonic acid (A.A.). This acid is rapidly converted by other enzymes. In the clotting process it gives rise to a chemical called Prostacyclin and to Thromboxane (TxA2). These two compounds have totally different effects. Prostacyclin prevents cells clumping together and opens or dilates blood vessels. TxA2 on the other hand is the most potent inducer of platelet release and aggregation known. The initial control of clotting is the result of a balance between stimulation and inhibition of platelets clumping together. The subsequent transformation of the platelet plug into a clot occurs as a result of the imbalance between pro-clotting and anticlotting factors in blood.

Platelets

This process is fine and also necessary when you suffer a wound. It is a totally different kettle of fish when the platelets start to bunch together when there is no wound. Normally blood should not be sticky but some studies have shown that victims of heart attacks have blood which is more than 4 times stickier than normal and if you look at their blood under a microscope you can see their platelets sticking together and also to the walls of their arteries.

What causes platelets to begin this sticking together without a wound? Normally the platelets are flowing through arteries and veins in contact with a number of chemicals which help it keep its disc or plate shape. But if it comes in contact with a lump of cholesterol or the wall of an artery which has been damaged by cholesterol sludge then chemicals from the cells of the artery wall can trigger off a change in the shape of the platelet from a disc to a sphere. The platelets also develop little suction pads which help them stick together.

Platelet Activating Factor

One of the chemical triggers for this process is called Platelet Activating Factor or PAF and it has a key role to play in the story of Ginkgo because the ginkgolides actually block or "antagonise" PAF. PAF is formed by a whole range of cells found mainly in blood, e.g. white blood cells called eosinophils because they are stained by the dye eosin, by platelets themselves and also by the cells which line blood vessels. In addition to activating platelets to change shape and stick together, PAF also "switches" on most of the inflammatory cells in the body and starts a series of events related to inflammation. There are many events identical to those arising from PAF-induced inflammation which also occur when lack of oxygen causes cerebral ischaemia and the common link seems to be Arachidonic acid.

The brain damage arising from brain ischaemia results from a complex mixture ("cascade") of processes affecting blood flow, brain electrical activity, and various biochemical reactions and includes many interwoven vicious circles. Once blood flow through the brain falls below a critical minimum level there is energy failure, changes in the levels of sodium, potassium and calcium and oedema or swelling leading to cell damage. The accumulation of calcium appears to have a key role in the process leading to irreversible nerve cell damage and death. It seems to lead to the switching on of a series of events which are toxic to nerve tissue, e.g. the formation of lipid peroxides, the generation of free radicals and the activation of protein dissolving enzymes and of pathological genes.

The first two of these processes involves Arachidonic acid. This normally plays a key role in the transmission of electrical messages along nerve cells. When brain cells are injured or damaged through lack of oxygen, A.A. accumulates instead of being removed as soon as it is released in normal cells. A.A. becomes unbound from cell membrane and is rapidly converted into destructive metabolites which kill neurones (nerve cells).

We have already seen how A.A. is broken down in the clotting process. There are in fact two pathways by which the acid could be changed. These are named after the Enzyme or catalyst which speeds up the chemical changes. One is called the **Cyclooxygenase pathway** and this is the one involved in the clotting mechanism. The second is called the **Lipoxygenase pathway** and the end products are highly inflammatory leukotrienes. Impairment of this cascade of reactions leads to the formation of oxygen radicals – these are highly reactive, highly unstable molecules which lack a balance between the charges on their atoms. These radicals destroy brain cells by damaging their membrane coatings and upsetting normal electrical activity in the cell.

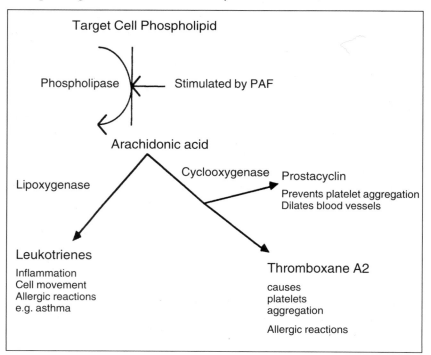

Ginkgo Flavones and Arachidonic Acid

The Ginkgo flavone glycosides described in Chapter 2 are believed to be one of the two major groups of active molecules in the leaves of the tree. It is believed that they could act in a number of possible ways which would reduce the harmful effects of the events described above on the brain. They could, for example, prevent the Arachidonic acid from being metabolised by inhibiting the two enzymes. Flavonoids in fact are well known lipoxygenase and cyclooxygenase inhibitors. Secondly they could affect the flow of calcium which appears to have a major influence on events. Finally, because they are anti-oxidants they can help remove the highly damaging reactive oxygen radicals by scavenging, by preventing their formation or by decomposing them. By this means Ginkgo can stimulate relaxation of blood vessels which have contracted, thus allowing more blood and oxygen to flow through to the affected areas and thereby reduce the long term damage caused by the ischaemia (figure 1).

Ginkgo was introduced in 1975 for the treatment of vascular diseases based on experiments which showed that it was able to lower the resistance to blood flow in arteries. However it was soon realised that the beneficial effects of the drug could not be totally due to its ability to regulate the contractability of the muscle tissue of the artery wall. It was clear from laboratory experiments that Ginkgo could protect animals from hypoxia and that it also had the ability to stimulate the synthesis of prostacyclin, which, as we have seen, prevents platelets sticking together and which also dilates blood vessels allowing more blood to flow through them.

The balance between thromboxane and prostacyclin is of vital importance in regulating clotting and other disturbances of blood circulation. This balance can be disturbed by lipid peroxides produced during the Cycloxygenase pathway which prevent cells producing prostacyclin. Ginkgo inhibits the formation of these peroxides and as a consequence stimulates prostacyclin synthesis. This can be shown in the laboratory by adding an extract of Ginkgo to strips of aorta (one of the big arteries which arise in the heart) and one can then measure the increase in the amount of prostacyclin produced.

By 1980 there were strong grounds for believing that the beneficial effect of Ginkgo was due to its ability to scavenge damaging free radicals and to prevent the formation of lipid peroxides. But it soon became clear from further experiments that other clinically important properties could not be explained by the aforementioned effects.

Brain Oedema

A number of scientists demonstrated that Ginkgo regulated energy levels in the brain during ischaemia and hypoxia. It was shown that Ginkgo

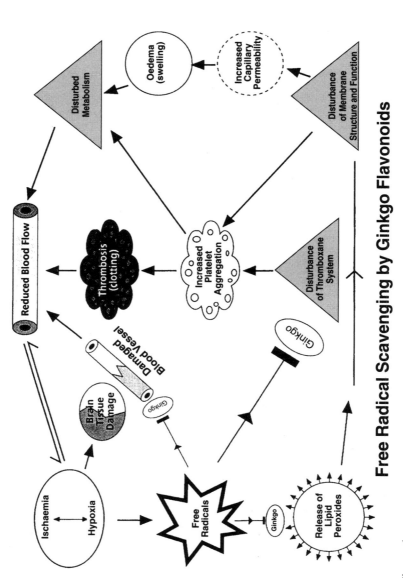

Free Radical Scavenging by Ginkgo Flavonoids

(adapted from S.S. Chatterjee)

Figure 1

given orally to animals could cure swelling (oedema) of the brain induced by a chemical triethyltin (TET). The significance of this laboratory finding stems from the fact that in humans this cerebral oedema is a major cause of lost body functions after a stroke particularly if the stroke results from internal bleeding or haemorrhage in the brain. The swelling of the brain with resulting compression causes a temporary loss of nerve conduction or communication between the individual cells. Apart from this oedema due to the squirting of blood from a burst blood vessel, brain ischaemia often also involves the formation of strong oedema which is one of the most serious complications of stroke and speeds up the fatal outcome. Experiments have consistently shown that Ginkgo prevents the full development of the brain cell-destroying oedema induced by TET in laboratory animals. Ginkgo not only reduces the elevated water and salts content of the swollen brain but it also has an effect on brain shape and appearance. Ginkgo maintains essential glucose and energy levels in situations where the brain is deprived of oxygen.

As knowledge of how Ginkgo protects the brain developed, people have accepted that this phenomenal plant has a multiplicity of actions. It was realised that, apart from the flavonoids, other chemicals from Ginkgo had a role to play. Systematic and detailed scientific studies led to the identification of the terpene bilobalide as an active constituent against the triethylin–induced toxicity. Removal of bilobalide from Ginkgo extracts always made them inactive.

Bilobalide

At an International Congress on Phytotherapy held in Munich in September 1992, attended by over 500 scientists and medical doctors, papers were presented describing the most up to date research on bilobalide. In one experiment bilobalide in doses up to 20mg per kg of bodyweight was administered to mice in which cerebral ischaemia had been produced by blocking a brain artery. The area of damaged brain tissue was carefully measured (infarct area). The bilobalide reduced the infarct area, with 5mg being the lowest effective dose. But, as Dr. Chatterjee told the same conference, the efficacy of the Ginkgo extract could not be predicted from the bilobalide content alone. Strange as it may seem, he found that addition of small inactive doses of bilobalide to certain inactive fractions of Ginkgo endowed them with high activity. In other words, these inactive chemicals could potentiate the action of bilobalide and, while bilobalide is a very effective compound, it is responsible for only one of the activities of interest. Other compounds also have their part to play.

Role of Ginkgolides

Since the early 1980's much attention has been focussed on the Ginkgolides which are known to be specific and potent antagonists of PAF. The belief that ginkogolides might also have a role to play came from a realisation that PAF. could be contributing to an aggravation of brain damage and oedema, particularly because it had been reported to increase the permeability of blood vessels thus allowing liquid to seep out into surrounding tissues. If Ginkgolides blocked PAF then they could prevent this happening. Experimental results indicate that PAF is likely to be one of the factors involved in brain oedema and that various Ginkgolides can prevent this. Studies in gerbils clearly show that Ginkgolides can inhibit phospholipase activation which we have seen is a first step in cell damage, that the accumulation of water and salt in brain tissue is blocked and that blood flow through the brain is improved.

Further experiments on animal models of stroke have shown that there is excellent recovery when Ginkgolides are injected two hours after ischaemia. Improvement was measured according to the widely used test of brain damage resulting from stroke – the so-called Stroke Index. The Stroke Index progressively tended towards normality when Ginkgolide B (which is known to be the most active Ginkgolide) was administered.

According to Braquet and Hosford [1991] Ginkgolides improve cerebral metabolism and protect the brain against hypoxic damage and there is significant antagonism of cerebral ischaemia and of all of the biochemical damage associated with it. Such studies in animal models with the Ginkgolides have shown that PAF plays an important role in a whole variety of pathological conditions and not just in central nervous system disorders. Obviously compounds such as the Ginkgolides which antagonise PAF would have great potential for treating a wide range of human diseases in which PAF is implicated.

The story of Ginkgo has therefore been closely caught up in the PAF saga in recent years and this wonder plant continues to surprise medical science and also to point the way forward to new treatments for old diseases.

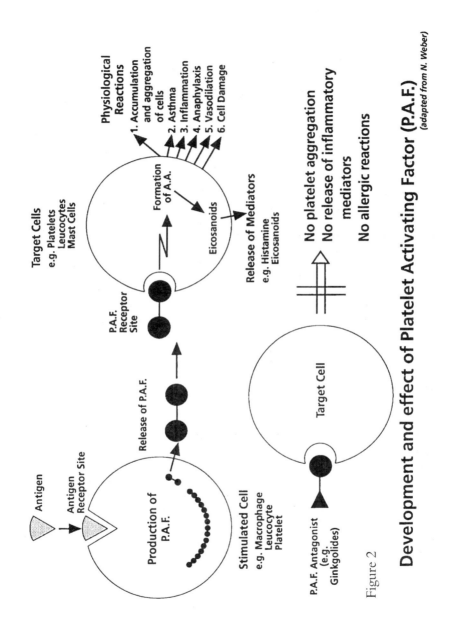

Figure 2

Development and effect of Platelet Activating Factor (P.A.F.)
(adapted from N. Weber)

4 | The Shock(ing) Story of Asthma and Transplant Rejection

Platelet Activating Factor (PAF) made only a brief appearance in Chapter 3 but for many people PAF is a real villain, having been implicated in diseases and conditions as varied as asthma, toxic shock, graft rejection, kidney disease and burn injuries.

PAF is produced by a range of inflammatory cells normally found in blood upon activation by an antigen or other stimulus which fits into a receptor site on an appropriate cell rather like the way a key fits into a lock. This sets up a sequence of events leading to the release of PAF from the stimulated cell (fig 2). The PAF then locks on to a specific binding site on a target cell thereby setting off a complex series of biochemical changes, some of which relate to blood clotting, e.g. platelet aggregation, and others relate to the release of Arachidonic acid (AA). Some cells release granular components including histamine and eicosanoids (twenty-carbon-containing molecules derived from AA) all of which are involved in various inflammatory processes including asthma, allergic reactions and the cell damage in the brain already referred to.

PAF and Asthma

Platelet activation is now known to be a feature of both allergic and non-allergic asthma. It is seen in asthmatics during tests or when the disease is exacerbated. Also platelets from asthmatics do not seem to last as long as normal because of this persistent activation. Asthma is a common disease characterised by an increased responsiveness of the airways [the trachea and bronchi] to a variety of stimuli which shows up as a widespread narrowing of those airways. Different triggers can cause such changes. Firstly there are allergens and viral infections which cause spasm of the bronchial smooth muscle [bronchospasm] and also hypersensitivity to various chemicals normally found in the body. Secondly there are triggers such as exercise, cold air and irritating dusts and gases which affect the severity of the disease by causing short-lived bronchial contractions.

Allergens are the most important in clinical practice with up to 80% of patients with asthma having allergies and as such labelled "atopic". When an allergen such as pollen or the house dust mite is applied to the skin of an atopic individual a classical triple response is seen within 15-60 minutes in the form of an acute wheal (a smooth slightly raised area of skin which is redder or paler than normal), a flare (a red outer zone of the wheal) followed some hours later by an area of swelling. In the lungs such an allergen causes an obstruction of the airways within 10-20 minutes which disappears spontaneously within 1-2 hours. Many asthmatics undergo a second episode of obstruction which can take up to 12 hours to disappear. This "late response" is associated with the infiltration of certain white blood cells (eosinophils) into lung tissue. This infiltration is stimulated by PAF which causes chemotaxis, i.e. it stimulates white blood cells to move into the surrounding tissue which in the case of asthma means into the pulmonary or lung tissue. These cells, so called because their contents can be stained and made visible under the microscope using the dye eosin, then release proteins which it is suggested damage the delicate lining of the trachea leading to hyperreactivity.

PAF is produced by several of the inflammatory cells involved in asthma. When injected into the skin of human volunteers it causes the wheal and flare response described above, followed in some cases by swelling. In the lungs PAF has been shown to be a very potent bronchoconstrictor in laboratory animals and in humans. In normal volunteers this acute bronchoconstriction lasts for about one hour. Different experiments have shown that PAF mimics many of the effects of an antigen both in skin tissue and in the lungs. Part of this harmful process is related to cell infiltration and part is due to our old friend Arachidonic acid.

When AA is changed by the lipoxygenase pathway it produces a series of very powerful inflammatory leukotrienes including a peptidoleukotriene which has the ability to cause spasms in the smooth muscles of the airways. Asthmatic patients are much more sensitive to peptidoleukotriene than normal patients. Human lung tissue and mast cells have the capacity to synthesise leukotrienes and peptidoleukotrienes have been shown to be released during asthmatic attacks or following provocation of allergic subjects by means of an antigen. These compounds are also found at higher than normal levels in osteoarthritis, in ulcerative colitis and in psoriasis. It seems reasonable to assume therefore that drugs which can block the effect of PAF on inflammatory cells could be of enormous value in asthma and other diseases.

PAF Antagonists

As fig 2 shows, PAF antagonists such as the Ginkgolides, which can fit into the PAF receptor site in place of the "real" PAF and jam up the works as it were, do not allow the release of Arachidonic acid and all its

27

dangerous relatives nor do they encourage platelets to migrate towards one another and to stick together. The search for PAF antagonists began shortly after it was first identified in 1972. One strategy was based on the study of natural products isolated from plants used in traditional medicine as anti-allergics. A number of such plants have produced useful compounds, Larix and Magnolia species, for example. *Ginkgo biloba* was an obvious target because the modern Chinese Pharmacopoeia describes it as good for the heart and lungs and the inhalation of a decoction of the leaves is recommended for asthma. Extracts of *Ginkgo biloba* were found to selectively antagonise PAF. Separation of the plant extract showed that the antagonist activity was confined to the non-flavonoid terpene fraction. Sophisticated separation techniques permitted the purification of the four Ginkgolides, A,B,C and M. Ginkgolide B was found to be the most potent antagonist. As a result the Ginkgolides have been subjected to hundreds of research studies. These show that Ginkgolides prevent platelet aggregation, clot formation and a variety of PAF induced chemical reactions.

Ginkgolides and Asthma

Ginkgolide B suppresses PAF induced eosinophil accumulation in the bronchial wall. In addition it has protective effects in PAF induced bronchoconstriction and airway hyperactivity in both animals and humans.

In guinea pigs the injection of PAF causes a fall in blood pressure and heart rate associated with bronchoconstriction of the airways. Ginkgolide B given to the guinea pigs either by mouth or by injection blocks both the cardiovascular impairment and the bronchoconstriction.

A commercially available mixture of the Ginkgolides A,B,C, in the proportions (40:40:20) was the first drug shown to be a potent PAF antagonist in humans and is currently undergoing clinical trials. According to a review by Braquet and Hosford published in 1991, doses up to 720mg as a single dose and 240mg/day for two weeks or 360mg/day for one week have been well tolerated by humans. The effectiveness of the drug in preventing various effects of PAF has been shown in human volunteers. In a skin test on atopic patients Ginkgo inhibited the infiltration of cells induced by a PAF challenge. In addition it also counteracted antigen-induced bronchoconstriction in asthmatic patients. Asthmatic patients treated with Ginkgolides require six times more allergen to provoke the same amount of bronchial response as those who did not receive the drug.

Ginkgolide mixture given by mouth or by inhalation alleviates the prolonged reduction in peak flow rates observed following exercise-induced asthma. Patients with mild to moderate asthma at five different centres in France (16 patients per centre) were given 240mg of ginkgolide mixture daily for four weeks in 1987. The drug caused a significant improvement in peak–flow variations compared to those given placebo drug, i.e. an inactive dummy drug.

Effects of Ginkgolides in Shock

Shock is characterised by generalised hypotension (low blood pressure) hypertension in the lungs, increased permeability (leakiness) of blood vessels, platelet activation and can frequently be fatal. Injection of PAF into animals mimics shock but Ginkgolide B can block the lethal effects produced by PAF. Ginkgolides provide significant protection both preventively and curatively against different types of shock, for example, salmonella endotoxic shock, septic shock caused by bacteria and shock caused by mycotoxins produced by fungi. At present clinical studies in humans are under way to evaluate the effectiveness of Ginkgolide B in different shock syndromes.

Ginkgolides and Burns

Clinical studies have shown both a Ginkgo extract and purified Ginkgolide B antagonise the high inflammatory response to burns which is characterised by increased production of leukotrienes and superoxide. Kidney function is also improved as is the survival rate. Here again ginkgo is being assessed in humans to investigate its potential usefulness.

Ginkgolides and Transplant Rejection

One of the problems associated with transplanted organs is that of acute rejection where cells called lymphocytes accumulate in the graft and if the rejection is not reversed the grafted organ can be irreversibly damaged. Three immunosuppressants are currently used either singly or combined in organ transplant patients. They are Cyclosporine, Azathioprine and Prednisone. These drugs possess serious side effects: Cyclosporine causes kidney damage and high blood pressure, Azathioprine depresses bone marrow and white blood cell production, while Prednisone promotes bone decomposition, cataracts and diabetes. Recent studies have shown that Ginkgolide B can inhibit the effects of PAF on lymphocyte production. The survival of rats with transplanted hearts is increased when Ginkgolide B is (combined with Cyclosporine and Azathioprine, although it does not have any immunosuppressant activity on its own. One of the possible advantages of using Ginkgolides is that the kidney damage caused by Cyclosporine is suppressed by them without changing the immunosuppressant activity of the drug. Intense research in this area reveals that PAF is involved in the kidney damage and that Ginkgolides could be a new drug in the reduction of the kidney damage caused by Cyclosporine.

Organ Preservation

Another aspect of the transplant dilemma is the problem of organ preservation because, with the exception of kidneys, no other organs, e.g. heart, liver, lung, pancreas, can be preserved for more than a few hours. The lungs are the most poorly preserved organs. According to Foegh et al (1989), the number of lungs available for transplantation in the U.S. should be the same as for transplanted kidneys, namely, about 9,000 per year but is only about 100 per year because of preservation problems. Organs are usually preserved in a perfusion fluid containing electrolytes (salts), sugars and other substances including compounds which prevent oxygen radical activity. Recently it was discovered that Ginkgolide B given to both the donor and recipient, as well as in the perfusion fluid, preserved lung function significantly better than in control animals. Obviously further trials will be needed to see if this treatment could be used for human transplant organs.

Human Studies – Immuno Stimulant

Experiments in experiment animals is one thing, clinical use in patients is another. However, the situation is encouraging because preliminary studies in man substantiate the animal studies. In a carefully controlled clinical trial, 18 healthy male volunteers were given a Ginkgolide mixture or a placebo for 15 days. There was a very strong improvement in immune status in the individuals given the Ginkgo mixture compared to the control group. This effect may explain the potentiation recorded when the Ginkgolide mixture is administered with Cyclosporine for the prevention of graft rejection [Braquet and Hosford 1991].

Ischaemic Heart Disorders

Other experimental studies with Ginkgolides show that they have a protective effect against damage to heart muscle when it is affected by lack of blood (ischaemia). Ginkgolide B protects the heart against ischaemia, against life-threatening arrhythmias (where the heart beats ineffectively) and markedly reduces infarct size. This drug appears to have enormous potential as a potent safe drug in the therapy of human ischaemic heart disorders.

Other Effects: Psoriasis and Multiple Sclerosis

Because PAF is implicated in so many different damaging conditions, it is not surprising that the Ginkgolides are under investigation as beneficial drugs in all PAF- related disorders. Indeed the Ginkgolides are themselves used as experimental tools to investigate the exact role of PAF in disease states because they so powerfully block the latter's effects. Among the areas currently under investigation are the use of Ginkgo in acute pancreatitis, gastrointestinal ulceration, eye diseases, animal models of multiple sclerosis and inflammatory skin conditions such as psoriasis. In psoriasis the drug Dithranol applied to the skin is widely used. However it has an irritating effect which limits its use and the resulting inflammation is difficult to treat with common anti-inflammatory agents. An ointment containing Ginkgolide B was tested in healthy human volunteers and it suppressed the dermatitis caused by Dithranol, particularly when it was applied before the Dithranol treatment. There have also been some preliminary studies of Ginkgolide B in the treatment of Multiple Sclerosis (MS) which showed an improvement in neurological scores shortly after treatment had started. Obviously more detailed controlled studies are needed to establish if Ginkgolide or indeed Ginkgo has definite benefits for MS patients, but it would not be surprising if Ginkgo was of help, given its undoubted ability to improve oxygenation of the brain.

It is clear from the huge number of laboratory and medical studies that the Ginkgolides have enormous potential as new drugs for the treatment and prevention of many debilitating, painful and life-threatening diseases. There is little doubt that much of that potential will be fulfilled, but it is the present use of Ginkgo which is of more immediate interest and concern-to many people.

5 | But does it really work?

Medicines based on *Ginkgo biloba* are among the drugs most frequently prescribed by family doctors in Germany and France. In Germany in 1988 more than 5 million prescriptions for Ginkgo preparations were written and the total market is put at about $500 million per year. Sophisticated scientific studies of the constituents of Ginkgo leaves cannot explain on their own the popularity of these medicines. It is necessary nowadays to show that they are effective in humans and that they provide positive benefits without the risk of serious side effects.

The main medical indications for Ginkgo are in patients with disease of the peripheral blood vessels (i.e. in the legs), such as intermittent claudication and in the treatment of cerebral insufficiency. This latter is in fact an imprecise term that describes a collection of 12 symptoms in elderly patients: difficulties in concentrating and of memory, absent-mindedness, confusion, lack of energy; tiredness, decreased physical performance; depressed mood, anxiety, dizziness, tinnitus (ringing in the ears) and headaches. Most of these symptoms are associated with decreased cerebral circulation, many, as we have seen in Chapter 3, are considered early symptoms of either M.I.D. or degenerative dementia. Often, however, no explanation can be found, but many of the symptoms are clearly due to processes in the brain upon which Ginkgo and its various components have been shown to have preventive and curative effects.

Laboratory studies using the flavonoids, bilobalide and the ginkgolides, can provide valuable information but modern medicine demands that the benefits of a drug be shown in double blind randomised clinical trials. Double blinded means that neither the patient nor the doctor doing the tests knows whether the product administered is the test drug or an inactive dummy drug prepared to be identical to the test product [the placebo]. Patients are then randomly allocated to receive either the treatment or the placebo. The whole idea is to ensure that no bias affects the result and that any effects seen are genuinely due to the drug treatment and are not just due to chance.

Studies with Human Volunteers

Many of the early studies with Ginkgo were carried out using healthy human volunteers. In one study performed in what was than West Germany, 6 young volunteers received either a dose of *Ginkgo biloba* extract standardised to contain 25% of flavonoids or a placebo. This study showed a clear dose-related effect of the Ginkgo on vigilance as monitored by using an electroencephalogram [E.E.G.] to measure electrical activity in the brain. In 1984 Hindmarch from the Psychology Department of the University of Leeds gave three different doses [120, 240, 600mg] of Ginkgo extract or a placebo to eight healthy female volunteers in a randomised double blind crossover trial [a crossover trial is one where participants are alternately given the test drug and the placebo with a week free from treatment in between to allow a "washout" of the system]. One hour after treatment, subjects completed a battery of psychological tests including reaction and memory tests. Memory as assessed using the Sternberg technique, was found to be significantly improved following 600mg of Ginkgo compared to placebo. Hindmarch concluded that there was a specific action on central cognitive processes and he went on to say that the data suggest a potential use for Ginkgo in the treatment of patients suffering from senile or pre-senile dementia in which impairment of memory function is a prevailing characteristic [Subhan and Hindmarch 1984].

In the following year Schaffler and Reeh conducted another double blind clinical trial on healthy subjects. After 14 days treatment with Ginkgo the subjects were tested for efficiency while they were in a state of hypoxia induced by inhaling a mixture of oxygen and nitrogen. The results obtained support the belief that Ginkgo had a protective effect against the hypoxia resulting from cerebrovascular insufficiency.

In 1988 Warburton reviewed the results of 20 clinical studies including two double blind crossover studies; nine double blind studies, eight open studies [where both doctor and patient knew the identity of the medicine] and one open multi-centre trial. Most of the studies used 120mg of Ginkgo extract per day giving 30mg of flavonoids and 7.2mg of terpene lactones [ginkgolides and bilobalide] per day, although some studies used up to 360mg per day. Warburton concluded that many categories of elderly patients could benefit from Ginkgo, particularly those with dementias and those with decreased intellectual function associated with depressed states given the positive effect on mood. Interestingly, at the International Conference on Phytotherapy in Munich, September 1992, Stocksmeier and Eberlein from the Medical Faculty of the University of Mainz, Germany, studied the effect of Ginkgo on the depressive mood of patients over a 3 month period. At the end of the study there was a statistically significant reduction in depressive symptoms in the patients given Ginkgo compared to those given placebo.

There have been over 40 clinical trials performed using ginkgo to treat cerebral insufficiency. Only one trial in patients with dementia of vascular origin reported negative results although some critics of Ginkgo use maintain that there is no evidence that it is effective. However two Dutch medical scientists from the University of Limburg in Maastricht have carried out a critical review of all of the clinical trials performed on Ginkgo for cerebral insufficiency and for intermittent claudication

Ginkgo and Intermittent Claudication

Intermittent claudication is a condition which affects the blood vessels of the legs particularly. It is characterised by the absence of pain or discomfort in a limb when at rest followed by the commencement of pain and weakness after walking has begun, the intensification of the pain until walking becomes next to impossible and the disappearance of the symptoms after a period of rest. It is largely due to the blockage of arteries in the limbs.

Early studies with Ginkgo showed that it could have benefits in this type of disease by influencing the distance walked without pain and by causing a dilation of peripheral blood vessels. For example, Sorbini in 1973 observed an improvement in 72% of patients with circulatory problems in their lower limbs, and this improvement was maintained three years later. In 1976 Natali and Cristol treated 50 patients with a success rate of 82%. For some patients the maximum walking distance increased by 40%.

According to Kleijnen and Knipschild from the University of Limburg only two of the fifteen trials of Ginkgo for this condition are of an acceptable standard. A number of the eight German and five French trials were flawed they said because the number of patients was too small or the trial was poorly designed. One of the best trials was that performed by Bauer who treated 44 patients with Ginkgo and 35 with placebo over a six-month period. Bauer measured the distance which could be walked without pain, the maximum distance and also the actual flow of blood through the very small capillary blood vessels of the limbs. At the end of six months the improvement was statistically significant. For example the walking distance increased from 112 to 222 metres on Ginkgo, compared to 145 to 176 metres in patients on placebo. The other trial showed that patients who had limb pains even at rest, were improved, after infusions of Ginkgo extract for 8 days. The patients were asked to rate their pain on a scale of 1-100; those given Ginkgo reported that their pain level dropped from 61 to 30 while those on placebo showed a decrease from 51 to 39.

Kleijnen and Knipschild have published their reviews of Ginkgo research in the world renowned medical journal, *The Lancet*, and in the *British Journal of Clinical Pharmacology*. In their November 1992 Drug Profile of *Ginkgo biloba*, published in *The Lancet*, they note that further evidence for efficacy is needed in the case of intermittent claudication but that in their opinion this is the most promising indication apart from cerebral insufficiency.

In what is probably a coincidental response to this comment, two separate meta-analyses of the clinical trials of Ginkgo in peripheral arterial disease were published in 1992. Meta-analysis, for those who are, like the present author, mathematically challenged, is a sophisticated statistical tool which allows experts to summarise the results of a number of different clinical trials of a particular drug or medical treatment.

One of the meta-analysis was published in the highly regarded journal *Drug Research* and included five placebo controlled trials. In each study effectiveness was measured as an increase in pain-free walking distance on a standard treadmill. The results of the meta-analysis highlighted a real and significant effect by Ginkgo preparations compared to placebo. In the second study the effects of ginkgo extract were compared with the synthetic drug pentoxifylline (Trental®) prescribed by doctors in

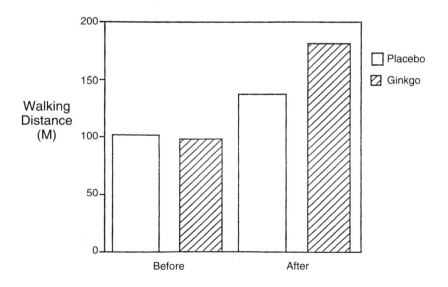

Figure 3

peripheral vascular disease including intermittent claudication. In this analysis some of the trials were ones included earlier but two were conducted in 1990. On average Ginkgo was found to give a 45% increase in pain-free walking distance compared to placebo in this meta analysis as shown in figure 3. The corresponding value for Trental® was a 57% increase in walking distance.

It seems that the value of Ginkgo preparations for intermittent claudication is now beyond reasonable doubt and due to its lack of side effects it is probably superior to other treatments.

Vertigo and Sudden Deafness

A number of earlier studies had indicated that Ginkgo may be of benefit in patients with vertigo, tinnitus and deafness of sudden onset. Studies conducted in the mid 1980's found that high doses of Ginkgo extract were superior to a number of synthetic drugs (e.g. piracetam) used to treat vertigo, sudden deafness and strokes.

A 1994 study compared Ginkgo with the preparation Praxilene® which contains the drug naftidrofuryl and which is prescribed in peripheral and cerebrovascular disorders. 80 patients with sudden loss of hearing were tested. Analysis of the hearing tests showed that after one week 40% of patients in each group had a complete remission of their deafness probably due to a spontaneous recovery. After three weeks the authors felt that Ginkgo was slightly superior to the Praxilene® and preferred the Ginkgo because it was without side effects, whereas some patients on Praxilene® reported headaches and sleep disturbances.

Pre-menstrual Syndrome

An early study of the possible benefit of a Ginkgo extract in cases of water and sodium retention associated with the menstrual cycle in young women, was performed in 1986 and indicated that oral treatment over a period of six months was beneficial in the small number of patients studied. In 1993 a French study found that Ginkgo extract was beneficial in dealing with some of the symptoms of the Pre Menstrual Syndrome [PMS]. This was a much larger study involving 165 women aged between 18 and 45 who received either Ginkgo tablets or a placebo. Changes in symptoms were evaluated by both the patients and their doctors without either knowing whether they were in the Ginkgo or placebo groups. While there was the expected sizeable placebo effect which occurs in any PMS study, those women on the ginkgo treatment still reported a significant improvement compared to placebo for symptoms such as breast tenderness and breast pain on palpation by the doctor.

For example, the number of women who did not experience breast tenderness after Ginkgo treatment over 2 menstrual cycles increased from 2 up to 20 compared to an increase from 8 up to 15 in the placebo group. There were also noticeable improvements in symptoms such as water retention (oedema), headaches, anxiety and depression but there was no statistical significance between treatment and placebo groups in these cases. Ginkgo has also been used successfully to treat cramps arising from uterine fibroids.

Ginkgo and Subarachnoid Haemorrhage

Haemorrhage from a ruptured blood vessel within the brain often causes difficulties with attention, memory, as well as feelings of illness, tiredness, anxiety and depression. The results of a study in 50 patients who had brain surgery for this condition was reported in 1993. The study was carried out as a typical medical study using one group given an inactive placebo and the other given tablets containing a Ginkgo extract of defined composition. As usual the test was performed double blind. After 12 weeks of treatment the two groups were subjected to an examination of attention span and of short term memory. The Ginkgo group showed a statistically significant improvement in reaction time. The number of errors in the reaction test was reduced by 65% in the Ginkgo group compared to a 2% reduction in the placebo group. There was also a significant improvement in verbal short term memory and selective attention in the group treated with Ginkgo.

Ginkgo and Cerebral Insufficiency

According to the 1992 review by Kleijnen and Knipschild, 40 controlled trials of ginkgo for cerebral insufficiency were performed between 1966 and 1991. Twenty studies were performed in Germany, 15 in France, 3 in Italy and 2 in the U.K. Using their system of evaluating the clinical trials, eight were deemed to be of acceptable quality. As in the case of intermittent claudication, the other trials had small numbers of patients, some did not describe the patient characteristics in sufficient detail or the effect measured was inadequate. They then compared the best Ginkgo trials with those for a drug called Co-dergocrine, obtained semi-synthetically from Ergot of Rye and which is a known vasodilator and metabolic enhancer and which has helped some Alzheimers patients in terms of blood flow to their brains and occasional improvement of mood and memory capacity. They concluded that the best trials of each product were of the same quality. In other words, the clinical medical evidence for Ginkgo is similar to that of a registered medicine for the same conditions. In fact one of the Ginkgo trials made a direct comparison of

Ginkgo and dihydroergotoxine in patients aged between 55 and 85 years old with symptoms such as dizziness, memory and concentration problems, headaches and depressed mood. After 6 weeks both groups showed improvements with no differences between the two drugs.

High Quality Clinical Trials

Among the trials listed by Kleijnen and Knipschild as being among the six best is that conducted by Meyer in 1986 in which 58 patients were given Ginkgo and 45 given placebo for 3 months and then followed up for 13 months. The average age of the patients was 50 years and they had all complained of tinnitus, dizziness and hearing impairment lasting 4-5 months. An improvement or total cure was found after an average of 70 days in patients treated with Ginkgo compared to 119 days in patients treated with placebo.

Taillander et al treated 210 patients [average age 82 years] with symptoms such as dizziness, tinnitus, headaches, lack of energy and difficulties in concentration and memory with Ginkgo extract or placebo on a daily basis for 12 months. They used a Standard Scale [EACG] for the clinical assessment of geriatric patients consisting of 17 items scored on a 7 point scale. Differences were assessed between groups after 3, 6, 9 and 12 months. After one month the difference in improvement between Ginkgo and placebo groups was 10/4%; after 12 months 17/8%. The small though clinically relevant effects are likely due to the very high age of the patients in this trial.

In the same year Haguenauer and co-workers investigated the benefits of Ginkgo extract [160mg] or placebo daily for three months in 70 patients with an average age of 50 years who had presented with a vertigo-like syndrome with associated tinnitus, headaches, nausea and loss of hearing. After 3 months 47% of the patients given Ginkgo reported that their symptoms had disappeared whereas only 18% of those on placebo reported an improvement.

More recently Vorberg and his group administered a standardised Ginkgo extract to 100 patients [average age 70] daily for 12 weeks. At the end of that time, improvements from baseline were:

		Gingko / Placebo
(i)	for difficulties in concentrating	54/19%
(ii)	memory	52/17%
(iii)	anxiety	48/17%
(iv)	dizziness	61/23%
(v)	headaches	65/24%
(vi)	tinnitus	7/12%

Vorberg reported his findings in 1989. Two years later Brüchert headed a group from the Association of German General Practitioners who assessed the effectiveness of Ginkgo extract in a multi-centre trial involving 303 outpatients with cerebral insufficiency. The average age of each of the patients was 69 and the average duration of symptoms was 46 months. Eleven of the "Classical" twelve symptoms of cerebral insufficiency [with the exception of confusion] were present in 45% of the patients. 95% experienced difficulties with memory. One hundred and ten patients received Ginkgo and 99 received placebo for 12 weeks. Three assessments were recorded; by the patients themselves, by the doctors and finally each of the 11 symptoms was scored on a scale of 1-4 [most severe]. After 12 weeks, significant differences were noted for eight of the symptoms. In the patients' own assessment 83% of the Ginkgo group felt improved compared to 53% in the placebo group. According to the doctors, 71% of the patients given Ginkgo had improved over the 12 weeks compared to 32% of the patients on placebo.

The final trial was that reported by Schmidt and his colleagues who treated 99 out-patients [average age 59 years] who had been diagnosed as having cerebral insufficiency. The average duration of the symptoms was 26 months. 50 of the patients received Ginkgo daily for 12 weeks, while 49 were given placebo. The difference in improvement in the classical symptoms was used for the effect measurement. After 12 weeks, significant differences were found for eight of the 12 symptoms. 70% of the Ginkgo patients felt improved compared with only 14% of the placebo group. The doctors scored Ginkgo slightly higher because they reported that 72% of the patients given Ginkgo had improved while only 8% of placebo patients showed a similar improvement.

From their intensive analysis of all 40 trials Kleijnen and Knipschild conclude that treatment with Ginkgo should last for at least 4-6 weeks before positive benefits are seen. They also conclude that Ginkgo can be given to patients with mild to moderate symptoms of cerebral insufficiency. It is not known whether the beneficial effects remained after treatment is stopped.

It is appropriate to conclude with a quotation from those two intrepid Dutch reviewers which appeared in the last paragraph in their article "Ginkgo biloba for cerebral insufficiency" in the *British Journal of Clinical Pharmacology*. In it they wrote *"another way to assess the evidence is to ask yourself whether you would take Ginkgo when you would have similar symptoms. Our answer would be affirmative: considering that there appear to be no clear side effects we both might try it."* So would I!

6 | Safe and Harmless?

When a medicinal plant has the powerful effects ascribed to Ginkgo and when it has so many potential uses, there is the feeling that there has to be a downside – some lurking fear of toxicity or side effects.

In fact, with the exception of the fleshy fruit and the seeds, Ginkgo and the medicinal products manufactured from it is remarkably safe. As has been described in earlier chapters, the outer fleshy seed layer has been known as a skin irritant for centuries. Contact with this outer layer can produce dermatitis resulting in oedema, erythemal reddening of the skin, papules and itchy blisters which disappear after about 10 days. If this fleshy layer is actually eaten, then one can get dermatitis of the sensitive mucous membranes of the mouth. The active allergens appear to be ginkgolic acid and bilobol [a phenolic compound totally different from the beneficial bilobalide] which are known to cross react with similar compounds from the Poison Ivy and from the Cashew Nut.

According to a recent review by Huh and Staba (1992) there have been no reports of toxic reactions to the Ginkgo flavonoids and ginkgolides. There appears to be no acute toxicity when tested orally in rats and mice. Toxicity is low when extracts of the leaves are injected either intravenously or into the peritoneum of laboratory animals. Staba however notes that toxicity to the seeds was reported in a 14th century herbal which referred to "ginnan" food poisoning. This seems to be due to an anti-vitamin B6 effect.

Many of the clinical trials of Ginkgo have taken note of any adverse reactions and to quote the most recent authoritative overview and critical appraisal of these trials *"no serious side effects have been noted in any trial and, if present, side effects were no different from those in Patients treated with placebo"* (Kleijnen and Knipschild, *Lancet*. Nov. 1992).

For instance, in his 1985 study, Vorberg tested Ginkgo extract on 112 patients and found in only a few cases that there were slight gastric symptoms at the start of treatment but these disappeared as treatment continued over a period of a year. Blood pressure and heart rate, blood lipids and cholesterol levels remained unchanged in all the patients.

Safety studies have also been performed on a mixture of Ginkgolides A,B,C, using healthy volunteers to whom doses ranging from 20-120mg were given. There were no effects on blood pressure, pulse, ECG and laboratory parameters.

In 1987 Barnes and co-workers from Kings College, London, administered the same mixture to 6 healthy human volunteers. One subject complained of drowsiness for 2 hours after taking 120mg of the mixture. Blood, liver and kidney tests remained normal when measured two hours after the ginkgolide capsules were taken.

In 1988 Warburton reviewed the results of 20 clinical studies and indicated that Ginkgo was devoid of side effects except for minor gastric problems. He also reported on a major study of 2,855 patients in which 3.7% reported gastric disturbances. Other very rare side effects included headache, dizziness and vertigo.

In an 1989 study of 8,505 patients two German researchers reported the total incidence of adverse effects to be a very low 0.4% with tummy upsets the most common at 0.1%.

More recently [1991] in a study by the Fachverband Deutscher Allgemeinarzte [Association of General Practitioners of Germany], using 150mg of Ginkgo daily in 303 patients, 16 adverse experiences were reported in the group given Ginkgo compared to 32 in the placebo group. More patients dosed with Ginkgo had headaches [4 Ginkgo to 1 placebo], burning eyes [1:0], and breathlessness [1:0]. In the same year a huge trial involving 10,815 patients was reported in Germany, with less than 1.7% of the patients [183 in all] reporting any type of side effect. The typical side effect was a gastric upset such as diarrhoea, nausea, indigestion, while some patients had headaches, ten patients in all had allergic reactions.

Another 1991 compilation evaluated the adverse effects which occurred during 44 clinical trials. In all 9,772 patients were treated with Ginkgo products and 51 adverse events were recorded. Again gastric effects were the major problem (21 patients followed by 7 patients with headache and 6 with dizziness). Laboratory studies have also demonstrated that Ginkgo is an extremely safe drug. Indeed it was not possible to determine a lethal dose because it was so non-toxic. Studies have also confirmed that Ginkgo does not damage the liver or kidneys nor does it have any effect in tests for mutagenicity which are used to predict possible cancer-inducing risks.

It is not surprising therefore that all of the scientists and clinicians who have studied Ginkgo medicines conclude that there is a very very low risk associated with products containing this plant. Given that those most likely to benefit from Ginkgo therapy are the elderly [who are known to use more medicines than other age group] it is also very reassuring that there are no known interactions with other drugs.

7 | And Finally

The importance of Ginkgo as a medicine is directly linked to the increasing number of elderly people in advanced societies. Unfortunately for many, the prospect of a longer life brings with it the increased risk of cerebrovascular disease. In addition to being a major cause of death [third after cancer and heart disease], it is the major cause of handicap in adults. One source estimates that approximately 500,000 people in the U.K. are incapacitated at present because of the effect of cerebral ischaemia on nerve cells.

Ginkgo can work wonders for such patients, improving their quality of life, reducing confusion, memory loss and associated symptoms. But is that the end of the story? Is there nothing left to say or to discover about this venerable tree? Can we truthfully say that the mystery which began with the first tentative stirrings of the fan-shaped bilobed leaves above ground, all those millions of years ago has been solved by the sophisticated scientific and medical studies of today's high tech. world?

I doubt that technological man can be so presumptuous as to boast that he knows all there is to know about this fascinating plant. There are still clinical studies to perform and there are still secrets to be unravelled.

One still unresolved mystery is that of the active chemicals from the tree. One Australian medical scientist, in the course of a review of a book on Ginkgo, wrote that as a pharmacologist he would prefer to see the isolation of the most active constituents, optimisation of their potency and recombination to provide a superior therapeutic product. While this classical approach has given us many highly esteemed drugs from nature [morphine, digoxin, vincristine, artemisinin, taxol] it is not relevant to Ginkgo. This approach begs the question – what are the active constituents? We have seen the spotlight rest in turn on the flavonoids, on bilobalide and on the ginkgolides. These latter of course hold out the promise of becoming major new treatments for a range of inflammatory disease and are very much drugs of the future but the story does not end with them.

We know that there are substances in Ginkgo which of themselves have no activity but which can increase the activity of bilobalide. Wouldn't it be foolish to discard them in our search for the elusive "active" principle?

The November 1992 issue of the *Journal of Pharmacy and Pharmacology* adds fuel to the controversy because it reports an effect of Ginkgo on the uptake of a key neurotransmitter by nerve cells due not to the ginkgolides nor bilobalide but to the flavonoid fraction. This increased uptake [which is predictive of an anti-depressant effect] was surprisingly not caused by the most prominent flavonoid and the authors state that other flavonoids or *other substances* [my emphasis] must be involved.

It is easy therefore to agree with Professor E. Ernst of the Physical Medicine Clinic, Munich University, when he says that while the benefits of *Ginkgo biloba* have been shown clearly, there is still a lot remaining to be done. He goes on to point out that the multiplicity of its effects are due to its chemical complexity. As to whether the search for "**the**" active constituent in this most ancient yet novel of medicinal plants is necessary, Ernst states "nature made an adequate natural blend for therapeutic benefit". To which I add − let us make the most of it!

Background Information and Further Reading

There have been many scientific studies, articles and books written about Ginkgo. In the preparation of this book a number have been found to be most useful and informative. They are listed below.

* Ginkgolides – Chemistry, Biology, Pharmacology and Clinical Perspectives.Vol. 1. P. Braquet [Ed.] 1988. J.R. Prous Barcelona.
* Ginkgolides – Chemistry, Biology, Pharmacology and Clinical Perspectives. Vol.2. P. Braquet (Ed.) J.R. Prous Barcelona 1989.
* Effect of Ginkgo Biloba extract on organic cerebral impairment. A. Agnoli et al. John Libbey Eurotext Ltd. 1985.
* The Ginkgolides: potent platelet activating factor antagonists isolated from Ginkgo Biloba L: Chemistry, Pharmacology and Clinical applications. P. Braquet (Institut Henri Beaufour, Le Plessis – Robinson France). Drugs of the Future 12 643-639.1987.
* Ethnopharmacology and the development of natural PAF antagonists as therapeutic agents. P . Braquet and D. Hosford. *Journal of Ethnopharmacology* 32 135-149 1991.
* Quality of Ginkgo preparations. O. Sticher. *Planta Medica*. 59. 2-11.1993.
* Ginkgo biloba. *American Botanical Council* 1991.
* Ginkgo biloba L. droque magique ou medicament moderne? R. Jasperson Schib. *Journal Suisse de Pharmacie*. 129 159-162 1991.
* Ginkgo biloba. Jos Kleijnen and Paul Knipschild. *The Lancet 340*. Nov. 1992 1136-1139.
* The Botany and Chemistry of Ginkgo biloba. L. Hoon Huh and E. John Staba. *Journal of Herbs, Spices and Medicinal Plants*. 1.91-124.1992.
* Ginkgo and people – A thousand years of interaction. Peter Del Tredici. *Arnoldia. 51* 2-151991.
* Ginkgo biloba for cerebral insufficiency. Jos Kleijnen and Paul Knipschild. *British Journal of Clinical Pharmacology 34* 352-358 1992.
* Neueste Forschungs ergebnisse zu Ginkgo biloba. *Munchener Medizinische Wochenschrift Spezial* Juni 1991. p. 1-13.
* Ginkgo biloba Extract (EGb.761): Pharmacological activities and clinical applications. F.V. De Feudis,. Elsevier Amsterdam 1991.
* Standardised Ginkgo Extract. Recent Research Part 1. *Mediherb Monitor no 11*. December 1994.
* Standardised Ginkgo Extract. Recent Research Part 2. *Mediherb Monitor no 13*. June 1995.
* When your loved one has Alzheimer's. David Carroll. Harper and Row New York 1989.
* Stroke – A Self Help Manual for Stroke Sufferers and their Relatives. R.M. Youngson. Clio Press Oxford 1988.
* Platelet Activating Factor – Ein Physiologisch Aktives Etherlipid N. Weber *Pharmazie in Unserer Zeit* **15** 107-117 1986.

8 | Index

OTHER BOOKS FROM AMBERWOOD PUBLISHING INCLUDE:

Aromatherapy − A Guide for Home Use by Christine Westwood. All you need to know about essential oils and using them. £1.99.

Aromatherapy − For Stress Management by Christine Westwood. Covering the use of essential oils for everyday stress-related problems. £2.99.

Aromatherapy − For Healthy Legs and Feet by Christine Westwood. A comprehensive guide to the use of essential oils for the treatment of legs and feet, including illustrated massage instructions. £2.99.

Plant Medicine − A Guide for Home Use by Charlotte Mitchell MNIMH. A guide to home use giving an insight into the wonderful healing qualities of plants. £2.99.

Woman Medicine − Vitex Agnus Castus by Simon Mills MA, FNIMH. The wonderful story of the herb that has been used for centuries in the treatment of women's problems. £2.99.

Ancient Medicine − Ginkgo Biloba by Dr Desmond Corrigan BSc(Pharms), MA, Phd, FLS, FPSI. Improved memory, circulation and concentration are associated in this book with medicine from this fascinating tree. £2.99.

Indian Medicine − The Immune System by Desmond Corrigan BSc(Pharms), MA, Phd, FLS, FPSI. An intriguing account of the history and science of the plant called Echinacea and its power to influence the immune system. £2.99.

Herbal First Aid by Andrew Chevallier BA, MNIMH. A beautifully clear reference book of natural remedies and general first aid in the home. £2.99.

Natural Taste − Herbal Teas, A Guide for Home Use by Andrew Chevallier BA, MNIMH. This beautifully illustrated book contains a comprehensive compendium of Herbal Teas giving information on how to make it, its benefits, history and folklore. £2.99.

Signs & Symptoms of Vitamin Deficiency by Dr Leonard Mervyn BSc, PhD, C.Chem, FRCS. A home guide for self diagnosis which explains and assesses Vitamin Therapy for the prevention of a wide variety of diseases and illnesses. £2.99.

Causes & Prevention of Vitamin Deficiency by Dr Leonard Mervyn BSc, PhD, C.Chem, FRCS. A home guide to the Vitamin content of foods and the depletion caused by cooking, storage and processing. It includes advice for those whose needs are increased due to lifestyle, illness etc. £2.99.

Eyecare Eyewear − For Better Vision by Mark Rossi Bsc, MBCO. A complete guide to eyecare and eyewear including an assessment of the types of spectacles and contact lenses available and the latest corrective surgical procedures. £3.99.